Your Hero

D1414662

Discover How Stroke Recovery Begins In Your Brain

Dr. Karen Malone PT, DPT

This book is not intended as medical or professional advice.

If you find this book helpful, please consider leaving a review at amazon.com. Help others find it and know that it is available!

Thank you!

This book is dedicated to the stroke survivors both near and far who I have had the privilege of working with over my entire career. I also dedicate this book to my previous students as far away as China who welcomed the opportunity to learn effective stroke rehabilitation techniques.

Above all I give thanks to God for all He has done in my life and in my heart. To Him be the glory!

Table of Contents

Table of Contents

Preface

This book is for anyone who wants to know a great place to start when developing a stroke rehabilitation program.

This is not a stroke exercise book nor a medical explanation of stroke.

This book is intended to be an eye opener. It is a book to help explain how the body moves when there has been no neurological injury.

Why consider these things? Because I believe stroke exercises, whatever kind is chosen, should be about helping stroke survivors function at their highest level. Rehabilitation should help open up new pathways for ongoing recovery. Learning how the body moved before the stroke gives direction in how movement needs to be regained.

I believe when it comes to regaining more normal function after a stroke...there is a Hero.

Introduction to the Author

Dr. Karen Malone PT, DPT is a Doctor of Physical Therapy and currently sees clients as a Mobile Physical Therapist in their home, office or community. Dr. Karen also offers computer-based online telehealth physical therapy consultations as a movement coach for wellness or for physical therapy evaluation and treatment.

She received her physical therapy degrees at the University of Illinois, Chicago, IL, and at the College of St Scholastica, Duluth, MN.

Dr. Karen is a single adoptive mom and lives in Saint Paul, MN, with her son, Silas, who is from China. She has been an international instructor in stroke rehabilitation with over 30 years of experience as a dedicated therapist to her patients and a trainer for both healthcare providers and caregivers. Her mission has been to advocate for the kind of stroke therapy that helps release the 'Hero' in the brain which leads to optimal recovery. The brain is responsible for creating what we recognize as normal movement. This in turn can lead to being able to participate in joyful activities at every level of stroke recovery.

Chapter 1

"Stroke 101"

What happens after a Stroke?

There are hundreds of thousands of people each year in the US who have strokes. Fortunately, there is more stroke education hitting the radio, newspapers and social media so that stroke symptoms are often recognized earlier and effective treatment can be promptly administered. An informed public is a prepared public!

Here are the signs you need to be aware of if you think someone around you is having a stroke. Prompt response can save lives, and in many cases, it can lessen the damaging effects of stroke. Remember the word, FAST.

FAST	
Face	Look for a drooping side of the mouth.
Arm	Look for one arm becoming weaker than the other or numbness.
Speech	Listen for slurred speech.
Time	Get medical attention as soon as possible even if you are not sure if someone is having a stroke. Some symptoms are subtle. Call 911.

After a stroke and the initial hospital intervention, the survivor and his family will have many questions about how to engage in the recovery process in order to reach the best outcome.

I have written this book to help those affected by stroke reach their goals. In order to do this, as a physical therapist, I want to walk with you into the past before the stroke occurred. If you are a stroke survivor, studying some things about normal movement will be extremely helpful in deciding your path forward. Finding exercises geared toward regaining those earlier movements will help you reclaim lost function due to a stroke.

As soon as physical therapy begins, I suggest that you communicate with your therapists about your personal goals.

Make sure that the therapy goals are not just to get you up out of bed and back home, but to work on the functional control of specific areas of the body and joints right from the start. This control of specific joints will not only relate to walking better but also enable you to return to a more functional life. The pot of gold at the end of your rainbow is regaining the best possible function!

These early days of rehab are the best days to reconnect your brain with key areas and joints of your body. As time goes on, this reconnection becomes more difficult, but not impossible. The brain will start soon after the stroke to try to move the arm and leg by using 'primitive' patterns of movement that will not be functional.

These are patterns that link each joint of a limb together into one movement, and cause the limb to move as a whole into odd positions. When this happens, the shoulder, elbow, wrist and hand all move into one of two major patterns, the extension pattern and flexor pattern.

This means that when the person tries to lift or use the limb each joint in the limb either bends up completely or jets out straight. Refer to the box below to better understand the difference between the abnormal flexor pattern response and the actual kind of movement needed to reach for a cup. The brain is sending the message to the arm that it wants to grasp the cup but the response can be very different depending on whether the brain's message can be divided up differently for each joint or if the brain is only able to send one message of total flexion. The movement begins in each case with bending the arm up in order to reach a cup on the table in front of the person. However, the flexor pattern will also include lifting the shoulder up toward the ear which is not a normal movement pattern.

Flexor pattern in the arm after a stroke.
Shoulder lifts and arm raises > elbow bends
> wrist bends > fingers bend. The whole arm
moves toward the trunk of the body.

Normal pattern used for reaching for a cup on a table.
Arm raises > elbow straightens > wrist is in neutral or bends back somewhat > fingers open. The arm is outstretched and the hand grasps the cup.

The abnormal flexor pattern does not allow for the arm control needed to first get the cup and then bring it to the mouth in order to drink from it. Therefore, the brain needs to be taught to first inhibit or prevent the abnormal movement pattern (shoulder lifting) and then taught to use normal movement patterns similar to those you were using right up to the time you had your stroke.

Normal movement patterns allow the joints to move independently of one another.

One key point I will make over and over in this book is that your injury was in your brain and though you see changes in parts of your body like your face, arm and leg, these areas are not injured.

I repeat. The injury was in your brain. It was not in your arm or leg. Therapy needs to be brain-focused and this means addressing the brain's ability to control the parts of your body that are not moving well.

Many people focus on the idea that the affected side of the body is just weak. However, at the time of brain injury your body did not first lose strength. It lost control.

The power station went down just like the lights go out in the house when power lines go down. If the lights go out in a house, no one goes around changing lightbulbs when they know the problem is the power source!

Due to the lack of brain control over the weeks that followed the stroke, you probably experienced the initial flaccid stage (low tone in the muscles). Perhaps your arm just lay beside you in the bed and you could not get it to move. When the flaccid stage ended, muscle tone in the body changed and you began to see movement.

If recovery of muscle tone took several weeks, some of your muscles lost strength from disuse but remember it is not because of muscle damage. As the brain heals it begins to be able to move some muscles in a limb and that is very encouraging.

Other muscles over time can become high in tone and in your case may have become tight making joints stiff and joints hard to straighten. Perhaps a hand is hard to open.

Generally speaking, our brain 'speaks' to the muscles telling them when to move, how to move and also when to relax. After a stroke, your muscles were left not 'hearing' the same message from your brain that they had heard for years before the stroke. Indeed, if your arm or leg could talk to you now they might say, "This is very weird! What am I hearing? What am I supposed to be doing?"

'Crazy talk' started to come down from the brain after the stroke which resulted in whole muscle patterns in your leg and arm unlike anything they did before.

When trying to lift the arm, the shoulder started to move up toward your ear! The elbow bent up and the wrist bent down. Your hand perhaps went into a fist.

That wasn't what you were hoping to see when you wanted to use your hand to drink from a cup. You knew something wasn't right! It may even have felt like your affected side was hijacked or had a mind of its own!

Now how can you stop these strange patterns from happening?

You must remember one thing. You moved very well for many years before your stroke and for this reason you have movement memory tucked in your brain. The extent of damage will affect how easily movement memory can be accessed and used by the brain.

No two strokes are the same. No two people have the same potential of recovery but maximizing that potential will be affected by the kind of exercise practiced and the brain's ability to message the body to perform functional movement.

It is possible in many cases to rediscover the correct brain messaging or a better message than what your muscles are hearing from your brain today! These messages have to run along new neural pathways.

These pathways need to be created and practiced to the highest level at which the brain can function today.

You have a Hero and your Hero is in your brain!

Understanding the Focus of this Book

In this book you will begin to understand that there is a process to developing a good stroke recovery plan.

We have to find ways to tap into the brain's best response during your daily experiences and functional activities. We are not just trying to evoke any kind of muscle movement. The movement needs to be useful and controlled.

I can't emphasize enough how much better you will move if you receive neuro or brain-focused therapy at this time.

Only addressing strength issues and neglecting joint control may hinder your brain from the ability to regain good function and good whole body movement.

Strength without control can appear more 'crazy' looking than functional. As an example, a gas pedal is not useful in a car if the steering is off! Strength and control of that strength (body and brain) must work together.

At the end of the day, learning to move in the most comfortable, balanced, coordinated and strong way will go far! Trust me! With good practice, your brain may be able to show you that it has these movement skills and movement memory reserved in millions of brain cells, not just in the actual cells that were damaged.

In addition, not all brain cells in the area of the injury have died. Some are damaged and will begin to heal. Some are affected by swelling that will resolve in time.

Think of pathways of communication leading from your brain to your body. After a stroke these neural pathways to the affected side of the body are working like an interstate highway 'spaghetti junction' trying to find the correct brain body connection.

There are many new connections being laid down in the brain itself and initially after a stroke these movement pathways may appear to be closed for repair.

Movement can begin to happen spontaneously as the brain swelling resolves and healing begins to take place! Limb movement may seem very weak and it might not be useful movement. Do not be discouraged when the simplest movements are difficult.

Remember two things during these initial days of healing:

1. Body Positioning

    Be mindful of how your body is positioned at rest during this vulnerable time when you cannot move yourself because this is crucial in determining how your muscles will 'wake up'. Good positioning can decrease the degree of high tone that will emerge. It will also keep your joints safe from injury because lying or sitting wrongly on your joints can cause damage and pain to those joints. Listen to therapists who instruct you on good bed and seating positions. When you need to change position, instruct those caring for you to never pull on your arm or neck or leg which can damage weak joints and cause pain.

2. The Type of Initial Active Movement

    How these neural pathways open up again will affect the traffic of messages to and from the brain. How the brain is retrained can have lasting effects on the way the whole system begins to function. Follow your therapist's instruction regarding the specific exercises and movements you should practice first. Later we will discuss certain keys to remember as you work to regain movement.

Let's find these new, good brain to body pathways as early as we can and do it in a way that will help you regain useful function!

I believe that an informed patient can become his or her own best advocate. When insurance stops paying for therapy, it will be you, not the therapist, that returns home to live your life. Because of this, make sure you and your therapist are working together on regaining the best quality of movement you need in order to do the kind of things you want and need to do more independently in the future.

Chapter 2

"The School of Normal Movement"

To better understand the effects of a stroke we must go back and take a look at how movement began in your life.

How did you learn to move the first time?

Why did we all learn to move our bodies as babies basically in the same way?

Perhaps at the beginning of this study we have more questions than we have answers, but as we take a closer look, we will begin to recognize the components that made up the normal movement patterns that were learned in the first years of our lives.

Babies and Movement

If anyone has been around a baby during the first half year of life, milestones are made seemingly every week. The baby loves movement whether experienced passively as he is handled by anyone who will pick him up or actively as he begins to realize and see more of the world around him.

Whole body movement will start and the child will squirm and wiggle during weeks of discovery fascinated that he has arms and legs that move!

Toys will be dangled around him enticing him to bat at them or kick them. He will begin to use wild, uncoordinated total patterns of movement. When the arm goes up, the elbow will bend and the hand will grasp. Eventually the baby will realize he can have an effect on the things in his 'world' when he sees his arm or leg accidentally make contact with an object near him and it moves! His brain will determine over time what movements are useful to reproduce the experience. He will begin to gain control over the muscles responsible for the movement he wants to create.

By attempting many different movements, the baby will begin to realize which movements bring him the most joy and satisfaction.

He will slowly learn to better control his arms, legs and eventually his entire body. His movement will become more purposeful and reliable over time.

He will learn how to maneuver each joint and how much force to use to create a desired experience. He will also learn which movements can more quickly get him what he wants.

Eventually while playing, he will discover that he can move his whole body to a different place on the floor.

Over time he will learn to scoot on his back or wiggle his body around in circles. Then one day after many days of trying, he will learn how to push himself over from his tummy to his back and then again to his tummy.

As he practices, he gets better at it and faster, too!

Over the next several months he will learn to push himself up to sit, fall over and do it again.

Deciding that some objects are much farther away than he can reach, the baby will learn to roll or to propel himself forward and backward on his tummy.

He will learn how to get up to play and crawl on his hands and knees. By the time he is about a year old he will be able to pull himself to standing and begin those precarious first steps!

The baby has been in the School of Normal Movement.

Though he may perform movement variations, his basic head, shoulder, trunk and pelvic movements will become more and more coordinated and useful in his life for changing his position and making him mobile. After that first year of life, his independence will finally be "won" and then the grown-ups in his life will be busy trying to keep up with him as he runs around on two feet in all directions!

As the child grows his movements will be refined and his coordination will improve. His brain will lay down pathways of communication to the body that will allow him to control the body well. This will happen through practice and repetition.

He will repeat the movements over and over again that are most energy efficient, most effective in attaining what he wants and that take the least amount of mental and physical effort.

The brain seeks ways it can conserve the body's energy when getting in and out of a bed or chair, as well as when moving the body across the floor such as when walking or crawling.

The amount of effort needed to accomplish a task will be noted in the brain and modifications will automatically be made.

The brain will reason that perhaps a movement would go better if the weight of the body were shifted further in one direction or if there was more rotation in the trunk at certain points during an activity.

As the child grows, he will try many different versions of movement to accomplish the same task and he will settle on what movement patterns work best!

Eventually the child will get good at skipping, jumping and even riding a bike!

Each new opportunity may offer new challenges, but the brain will base much of its ongoing study and mastery of movement over the first several years of life on the basic movement patterns previously learned and the natural balance reactions experienced as an infant.

Babies and toddlers learn something new every day through movement and become stronger and stronger in the process.

Motor development is happening as the baby practices purposeful movements. The movement and the purpose of the movement are being woven together in the brain so that eventually he is not focused on how to move the body but on what he hopes to accomplish.

Movement memory is being laid down in the brain.

Adult Movement

What influences how an adult changes positions in bed, gets out of a chair or climbs a ladder?

The answer is gravity and body mass. The baby had to deal with these and so does the adult, only the adult brain has mastered so many effective movement patterns that the movements now look smooth and easy.

Gravity is consistent and plays a big role in the way we move. Gravity is a force or push on our bodies here on earth, and there needs to be an adequate push back against gravity to create movement.

When getting off the floor, for example, our muscles create that push upward and the strength of that push depends on body mass.

How do we physically move our bodies?

Muscles are attached to bones and cross over our joints. When muscles contract, joints bend or straighten, turn or twist. The joint may even just be held still or fixed in one position.

We have over 650 large and small muscles working together. We have over 200 bones!

Ligaments hold our bones together at the joints. More than one muscle is responsible for performing a functional arm movement or a whole body movement.

Movement in one part of the body can affect how another part of the body moves. If I am sitting on the edge of a bed and bend my ear down to my shoulder it causes the weight of my body to shift to that side which makes muscles and joints move all the way down my spine.

When we move our bodies we use multiple muscles to move some joints and may at the same time use other muscles to stabilize other joints.

The combination results in this body of many parts ending up in a different position and ready to perform a desired activity or task!

In other words, movement of one part of the body may require holding firm or fixing another part of the body.

The stable part will give the moving part a place from which to move. For instance, the trunk holds firm so the arm can be raised overhead.

Another example of this is when we plant one foot on the ground while we move the other foot up on a step. We also hold our trunk fairly steady in order to be able to use our arm to swing a tennis racket or wash a window.

The Brain's Role in Movement Production

It is the brain that has the sole ability and responsibility for planning and executing the job of safely moving an entire body part or the entire body mass wherever it is needed in countless situations!

After a stroke, many people focus on just strengthening muscles on the affected side any way they can. They forget or don't know about the need to strengthen the muscles' connection to the movement control center of the body.

People can become discouraged because they wonder how the muscles on their affected side can be strengthened when these muscles aren't responding well?

It makes more sense to focus on *what* needs to connect up with the muscles in order for them to move well. It is the brain and its movement memory that first need a better connection to the muscles. Then these brain connections related to normal movement can become more readily accessible to the stroke survivor through repetitive practice.

A baby may start the process of movement by using his sheer muscle strength. However, the movement is jerky and uncoordinated.

Then as brain development continues the baby learns proper coordination (or body mechanics) to eventually assist the body to move effortlessly and safely all the way from lying on the floor to standing up on two feet and beyond!

Thankfully, the more accessible learned movements become, the more the child's efforts become less strenuous. These learned movements must include coordinating head, shoulders, trunk and pelvis in unison.

In addition, proper weight shift occurring throughout an activity will offer easier ways for the body to move. An example of this is getting your nose over your toes when moving from sit to stand which shifts the weight of the body toward the feet and off the bottom, thus allowing you to stand up more easily.

Movement becomes more and more fluid after it is learned so do not be discouraged during the learning phase of recovery.

Keep focusing on learning how to control muscles and joints rather than strengthening. The strength will come but you do not want strength without control.

Remember that learning is a process. Before a movement is learned, movement looks clumsy and awkward like when someone is learning to play tennis or ride a bike for the first time.

Summary

Human movement was meant to be fluid, not jerky, and the brain keeps practicing and refining the movement from babyhood to adulthood until those new moves look like they have been used for a lifetime! Practice will lead to fluid and coordinated movement.

These same previously learned movement patterns are most effective in producing functional movement after a stroke, and they should be a part of the stroke recovery program. Practicing the wrong movements over and over will not automatically lead to functional and satisfying movement.

Eventually, the child's brain and later the adult's brain will make countless movements every day with very little conscious thought, and most of the time with no thought at all!

These movements will change from feeling awkward to feeling familiar, from looking complex to looking simple.

The stroke survivor will need to really focus on normal movement patterns initially until some movements become more automatic again.

The Hero who makes that possible is in the brain!

Yes, *your* Hero is in your brain!

Chapter 3

"Balance 101"

In this chapter, we look at how a person keeps his body from falling over. Balance is the skill the brain has acquired to prevent falls. In the presence of gravity, balancing body mass is crucial for fall prevention.

Let's answer questions about balance and thus determine how much the Hero in your brain does to balance your body throughout your day and keep you safe! During stroke recovery, you will want to do the kind of exercises that will help your Hero improve your balance!

You might think that in order to learn balance a person must be sitting or standing a few feet off the ground. Perhaps walking on a balance beam or even on a street curb would offer an ideal place for balance to emerge.

Actually, just to get to either of those places a person already has to have some balance skill.

Rising up off the floor might be considered a good place to start to learn balance. After all, for this activity there isn't too far to fall!

Doesn't it take balance to stand up after getting down on the floor to look under the couch for your shoes? It does take balance but standing up from the floor is not where balance practice should start either!

Believe it or not, balance practice best begins on your back. That idea may seem strange because there is literally nowhere to fall! So how can balance be learned in a position where there is no risk of falling?

When Does Balance Happen?

Balance, as we all know, helps keep you from falling not just when you are standing still but also when you are in motion.

Balance occurs when someone is still and also when he is moving. It does not happen when the body is at rest such as when someone is lying relaxed on a bed or sitting completely supported in a chair.

Balance movements occur when something is trying to force the body into a different position or place and the body needs to resist or adjust itself to keep from falling.

Balance happens when someone decides he wants to change his position and it requires some kind of upward shift from a supporting surface (e.g., when climbing a ladder and even when rolling over in bed).

Balance also occurs when the body wants to start moving into a position or along a certain path and gravity or an external force resists the movement (e.g., trying to walk a dog along a path when the dog is pulling on the leash because he is trying to chase a cat across the yard or a child trying to walk up a slide at the park but keeps sliding back toward the ground).

Balance is essential to our daily lives and will affect our level of function.

Balancing Against Gravity

What about when someone is lying on a level floor? Are balance movements needed then? They are not needed if the body is at rest. As soon as the body begins to move away from the floor such as with rolling, balance reactions will emerge.

In order for you not to fall through the floor, the floor must push up on your feet as you stand on it. The force of gravity pushing you downward on the floor creates the force of the floor pushing you upward.

If you don't fall through the floor, then we say that the floor can bear your weight. Remember that gravity and your body mass are always present.

To move your body away from a supporting surface of a bed like when rolling, you must overcome gravity. You overcome gravity with continuous motion until the roll is complete. In other words, a person can roll over without stopping at any point.

The movement could be described as 'fluid movement'. Throughout the entire rolling process, the brain is producing the body's "fluid movement" as segments of the body are moving either independently (e.g., when the head is initially lifted up) or in unison with other segments of the body (e.g., when the arm and leg on one side of the body cross over in front of the body at the same time the trunk on that side of the body is shortening).

This concept helps us to understand why balance reactions can begin on the floor! As soon as the body starts to rise above the surface of the floor or bed, gravity will be pushing down and trying to put the body back into a position of resting on the supporting surface.

Balance happens because gravity is always working against the body's efforts to move against gravity. The body is pushing into gravity or being pushed by gravity.

Muscle and joint control created by the brain allows for the body's mass to move effectively in the presence of gravity. Strength will be required, but the actual muscle and joint control will steer the strength in the right direction and keep the body balanced.

Most of the time we are not moving in the direction of gravity's pull unless, for example, we are descending a flight of stairs or sitting down on a chair. If we are purely being moved downward by gravity with no muscle involvement, then we are falling.

Walking down the stairs is harder to do than falling down them because controlling your body as you descend the stairs requires balance. Sitting down in a chair without plopping also requires balance. Balance keeps us from falling.

If you are lying on the floor on your back and you want to lie on your tummy, you will need to overcome gravity that is pushing you into the floor. This will require muscle strength and coordinated movement. It will require movements associated with balance.

We know that rolling is easier to do with good muscle strength as well as the right coordination or control of various muscles at particular times throughout the rolling process. We realize this even more after a stroke when rolling is more difficult.

Balance Reactions

Balance reactions are directly related to the position of our center of gravity over our base of support. The base of support of our body is the area beneath the body's center of gravity. Muscle movements are used to maintain our center of gravity over our base of support and prevent a fall.

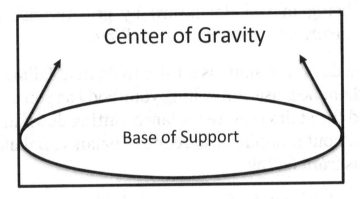

Our base of support can change. Spread the feet apart and the center of gravity has a larger area in which to move.

We feel stable with our feet apart and are not easily tipped over. Bring the feet together and the base of support is greatly reduced limiting the degree of movement in which our center of gravity can easily move.

We have to work harder to stay standing over a narrow or small base of support, particularly if we were pushed.

When the body's center of gravity gets close to the boundaries of the base of support and goes beyond the base of support, our balance reactions start to emerge.

Balance reactions occur when there are shifts in the position of the skeleton left and right or forward and back. These shifts can move the center of gravity beyond the base of support, but since we are not like a log, we have ways to compensate for excess movement in one direction by bending our joints.

For instance, as we sit down, when our hips move behind our base of support then our shoulders will move forward to counterbalance the backward tendency of the skeleton.

We can bend at the waist to move the shoulders forward. Because we did this, we can stay balanced over our base of support as we bend our knees and lower our body to the chair.

Balance is absolutely necessary for our mobility and stability, e.g., when walking to a chair or sitting on the edge of a bed.

Being strong is not the same as having balance. Even after a stroke, you may be strong in your legs and still not stand or walk well. Strength is not enough to help you balance over your base of support.

A good question about your balance during your stroke recovery process is, "Can you get yourself into a position such as standing, and can you stay or balance yourself there to do something useful or functional with your hands?"

Balance and Functional Exercises for Gaining Strength and Control

Here are some good questions to consider when developing a stroke recovery exercise and balance program.

How did the baby's brain first start to learn balance?

Was it by doing baby pushups and leg presses or by learning to control various muscles during a functional task? It was, for instance, when the baby was sitting on the floor reaching for a toy or when he was attempting to move his body closer to a desired object.

Were strength and control working together from the start to accomplish something specific? If so, then the brain will remember how to use an arm or leg along with the memory of the specific task.

The importance of incorporating a functional task early into therapy cannot be underestimated. Should stroke rehab initially be only about strengthening or should it also be about strengthening the body during coordination and balance activities geared toward accomplishing a meaningful task?

The baby did not learn balance by doing baby pushups and leg presses but rather the baby became stronger and more balanced while he was finding a way to get to a toy so that he could play.

Before a stroke, balance adjustments are made with ease and with subconscious thought. The brain stays consciously focused on the meaning or purpose of the task or activity at hand.

These tasks are often referred to as functional tasks. Examples include standing and showering, mopping a floor or mixing cake batter at the kitchen counter. A person is most motivated to move during a familiar task and the brain often associates specific coordinated movements with the memory of specific learned tasks. Here is another clue for developing an effective stroke rehabilitation program!

Balance and Sensation

Sensory input during therapy could include sitting on different kinds of surfaces like a firm chair, a soft bed or an air pillow. It could also mean standing in a crowd or walking through knee high water in a kid's pool.

Balance works by combining coordinated muscle movements throughout the body in response to sensory feedback that is going to the brain.

The brain may sense that the ground under the feet is not level and it makes adjustments to the skeleton by relaxing or contracting various muscles. This creates movement around a number of joints.

These movements or balance reactions are effective and successful in starting, maintaining, controlling and stopping the body that could otherwise fall.

By making balance adjustments the person can, for instance, continue to walk on the grass to the shed to get a rake or stand in the yard when watering the lawn.

Incorporating the body senses early into rehab is helpful in recovery. Sensation is an input message to the brain from the body. Muscle movement is due to the output message from the brain.

This kind of communication between what is sensed and what to do about it is happening all the time and helps a person stay balanced.

Balance is the coordinated work of the body using its senses like vision, spatial awareness or feeling different types of sensation (discomfort, pressure, slipping...) and then responding with changes in muscle length to close, open or stiffen a joint or joints in order to stabilize the body in one place or move the body or a part of the body to a different place.

I can try to balance on one foot on my kitchen floor or I can try to balance as I walk along a log. In both cases, I am getting sensory input from my surroundings and then responding with muscle action.

The ability to feel the arm or leg is necessary for good stroke recovery. It is very difficult to learn to move something that you cannot feel. Sensation is also necessary for good balance.

Balance and Motor Planning

In some instances, balance occurs when the brain responds to a change in the environment. For instance, when the sidewalk becomes uneven and the person's footing is not stable the body will need to make changes in order to prevent falling.

Balance movements may also be anticipated. This happens particularly when the brain plans to move the body through a movement it has previously mastered in order to accomplish a specific goal. In these situations, more than one thing is happening at the same time.

The brain plans how it will move in a balanced way to accomplish a task. The brain may start with the thought, "I want (something)" when it comes to planning a movement.

- "I want to relieve the uncomfortable pressure on my back from the bed."

- "I want to better position my hand to eat a piece of cake with my fork."

- "I want to position my body so I can drive my car."

- "I want to wash the dishes at the kitchen sink."

After one of these thoughts, the brain will motor plan and decide what part of the body needs to move, when it needs to move and how much effort will be needed from each muscle throughout the activity.

Motor planning for a previously learned activity will not need much time before the movement is executed.

The planned movement is then performed and at the same time the body and the body parts used for the task are kept balanced and coordinated during the activity. The person remains standing while washing the dishes.

Motor planning is required to perform a specific exercise in therapy such as a leg lift. However, incorporating a purposeful activity in therapy that requires motor planning and one that the brain has done in the past will help the brain more easily relearn motor planning skills for the actual tasks the person needs to be able to do.

Depending on a stroke survivor's abilities or skills, the therapist will know when to work on mat exercise and when to set up a specific functional activity that will require motor planning and balance.

In the therapy sessions I have with clients, I will often start with a mat exercise but end the session using the movements practiced during a functional task. Functional tasks should be a part of each session and take up more and more of the session time as the client improves.

Body balance is primarily being controlled at the neck, shoulders, trunk and pelvis. Each of these parts of the body are helping to initiate movement, maintain movement or stop a movement in order to stay balanced when standing still or walking.

We will see when we study certain keys to normal movement that these particular areas of the body majorly influence function.

They, likewise, can also help to influence how the Hero is able to automatically improve balance simply by making adjustments to each of these parts.

These parts of the body are leaders when it comes to balancing the body!

Balance Training on a Floor Mat or Mat Table

Let us look for a moment at the stroke recovery process as relates to balance. I would say that mat exercises in therapy are very key in order to work on isolated body movement. Head, shoulder, pelvis and hip control can be practiced easily and in a way that the client can see the part of the body as it moves.

You may have had therapy on a mat when the therapist passively moved your arm or leg. Perhaps you were not asked to try to move while lying on the mat. In my opinion, mat exercise is very useful and is not intended to be only passive, but should progress to assisted movement and then active movement.

As a therapist, I prefer to start working with every client on the mat table where the client can transition from sitting to lying down on his back as well as rolling from back to tummy. It is where I begin to best assess shoulder and hip movement, the degree of control at each joint and the client's ability to work against gravity.

Floor mat exercise is safe and effective in focusing the brain on joint movement without having to balance the body in a position higher off the floor. It removes any fear of falling or distraction because the person is already on the floor or mat.

For me, stroke therapy begins on the mat table or on a mat on the floor. In some cases, but not all client situations and conditions are appropriate, floor mat exercise will eventually lead to the therapist being able to facilitate all the movement needed for the client to be able to get himself to and from the floor using normal movement patterns. If it is not possible to get to the floor, then a mat table can offer many movement experiences necessary to relearn balance skills.

Summary

Can you see more clearly how balance can be learned when you are lying on your back on the floor with nowhere to fall? It will become even more clear as you continue to read!

The balance concepts in this chapter have helped to underscore the importance of targeting balance with functional skills, balance reactions, coordination and joint control after a stroke during rehabilitation.

Get a handle on ways to improve balance and you are well on your way to releasing your Hero.

Chapter 4

"Don't Forget Your Keys!"

What if after a stroke you were left to learn to move again using any movement possible? Do random movements lead to good balance and function? They most often do not.

There are some very specific movement components necessary in order to change or hold a position and in order to maintain balance at all times.

Learning these components is valuable after a stroke!

In other words, a poorly balanced body movement or the lack of a necessary movement at the right time can attribute to a fall. Gravity will not let us get away with poor body control.

The growing baby went from making frequent falls and balance failures to eventually no falls or balance failures. Most adults in their early years have very few falls and can go years without a fall.

The baby learned some proven principles of movement or "keys" necessary for good balance and successful movement.

What exactly did the baby learn that decreased the risk of a fall as he grew older?

Key #1	**Stabilization before mobilization**
Key #2	**Develop stability proximally to distally**
Key #3	**Normal movement requires normal tone**
Key #4	**Elongation on the weight bearing side with weight shift**

Key #1 Stabilization Before Mobilization

Stabilization and movement (mobility) often are happening at the same time in different parts of the body! Now that seems like a lot of work for the brain to do! What a Hero!

Examples:

- Stepping forward with one foot while standing on the other.

- Holding an arm away from the body before turning a doorknob with the hand to open a door.

A toddler who has learned to stand up from the floor will often stop or pause just as he reaches an upright position before he takes a step. Good movement happens from a place of stability. A bowler will stand holding the ball to her chest before initiating the swing of the arm and the steps to the line where the ball will be launched.

The shoulder and the hip need to be able to stabilize or maintain a position in order to give the hand or foot a better chance at being useful. (First, develop stability in the leg or arm before requiring it to do a movement.)

Imagine someone with a weak shoulder but a perfectly good hand carrying a laundry basket up the basement stairs. Or imagine someone with weak hips but perfectly good knees and ankles stepping up on a step in order to put away a piece of china in the cupboard.

This is why connecting the shoulder and hip up with a stable trunk can make a big difference. The Hero learned this key.

Adding this key early into stroke intervention can get someone further and faster in their recovery than if that person is immediately asked to sit and feed herself or walk down the hallway before she can sit or stand well. Poor stability means poorer quality of mobility.

It is important for the brain to be able to recognize when the body is actually in a midline position and when it is shifted left or right, forward or back from midline.

Stability in midline means a person can positioning herself in midline (she can find midline) and then hold the body in the midline position. Stability should precede the person practicing weight shifting the body side to side (mobility). Get the body stable in the middle and then get the body mobile!

Otherwise we will see a person, for instance, walking with her weight clearly over on one side and she may be wondering why walking is difficult. Stability before mobility will greatly affect safety, balance and even muscle tone.

Key #2 Develop Stability Proximally to Distally

Proximal means close to where the arm and leg attach to the trunk (shoulder and hip). Distal means farther down the limb (hand or foot). The hand is distal to the elbow and the foot is distal to the knee.

Key #2 ties in with Key #1 but is another aspect of how to progress stroke recovery and muscle balance.

If more control is wanted in a limb, then it is important to start gaining control proximally and then work on gaining better control distally. Start working with the shoulder and progress to the hand. This can happen during one therapy session.

Why is shoulder control important for hand use? Without being able to place the hand in a certain position by using a forward or an out to the side shoulder movement, the hand has less use or function.

Most things are not right up next to the body so the arms are used for reaching out and getting things! Likewise, without being able to control or hold the position of the hip whether it is holding it forward, extended backward or out to the side, the foot will be far less useful and helpful.

For example, holding the hip in flexion allows the foot to be placed on a step.

Key #3 **Normal Movement Requires Normal Tone**

Muscle tone is how tense the muscle is set even when it is at rest. It has nothing to do with temperature but think about the tone getting set like you preheat an oven.

Normal muscle tone keeps the part of the body ready to move but calm. (If it was temperature, it would not be too hot or too cool.) When there is normal tone in someone's muscle, then when someone else tries to lift that person's arm off the arm of a chair, the arm will move easily and seem light. It is like the arm almost anticipates where it should go and follows the suggestion of moving upward.

Why? It is because *the muscles are so ready and able to move!*

If there is too much tone in a limb, it cannot be lifted easily by another person but it feels stuck. Usually only the muscles on one side of the limb will be high tone. The lower tone muscles in that same limb do the opposite movement to the high tone muscles.

However, in the presence of high tone, these lower tone muscles cannot overpower or even balance out the pull of the high tone muscles and so the movement in the whole limb is limited.

The low tone muscles appear to be inactive and we see the limb move into the pattern of movement created only by the high tone muscles.

An example would be tense or high tone in the muscles that bend the elbow and do not allow the muscles that straighten the elbow to do any straightening motion. The tone in this case could be so tense that the person cannot move his arm at all and the arm feels locked in a bent position.

Often if there is movement in the arm after a stroke, it is in one direction because this movement is being performed by the high tone muscles in the arm. The arm can feel tight if someone else tries to move the arm in the opposite direction.

The arm can be painful due to the sustained contraction of those muscles. The limb does not feel light if another person tries to lift it up but can seem heavy and stiff.

If muscle tone is too low throughout the limb after a stroke, it is as if the muscles cannot 'hear' the brain's message to move and cannot 'pull themselves together' so to speak to respond. This is called flaccid muscle. The limb can feel heavy if another person tries to lift it and the limb just lies in one position as though lifeless.

Because tone begins in the brain we need to learn ways to decrease high tone and increase low tone. There are techniques that can help.

We also must consider that someone can have high tone that fluctuates from one set of muscles to another set of muscles in the arm. When the person tries to use his arm, it either bends all the way up or straightens all the way out.

A therapist can help address these challenges and try to help the person learn better control.

Abnormal tone (too high or too low) results in abnormal movement. Normal tone results in normal movement.

Change the tone and the movement can change, too!

Key #4 Elongation on the Weight Bearing Side with Weight Shift

The ability to weight shift well is crucial to normal movement.

Human body movement that is the easiest and most efficient requires weight shift. If a person sitting on the edge of the bed shifts her weight left, you may see the left side lengthens and the right side shortens.

The trunk side where the weight is shifted becomes 'longer' or stretches. The shoulder and pelvis on that side of the body move away from each other.

This is called elongation. It is the body's way of increasing stability on the weighted side as it unweights the opposite side in preparation to moving that opposite side.

In standing, a person will shift the body's mass to the left foot in order to take a step with the right foot. It is not possible to take a step with a foot if you are standing on it.

Stroke recovery should include weight shifting exercises before stepping exercises. Walking is more than just trying to move one foot forward. That foot must first be unweighted and the body needs to learn how to do that well.

Weight shifting to the left in standing should cause elongation on the left side of the trunk. The left shoulder will rise some and the left pelvis will drop. Thus, the distance between the two becomes 'longer'.

This weight shift left results in the right side becoming 'shorter'. The right shoulder and pelvis move toward each other and the trunk 'shortens' on that side.

Once the body is well set or balanced over the left foot, the right foot can easily be lifted up and moved forward. Poor weight shift to the left side will result in a shuffled right step, a shortened right step or could even result in a fall.

The person with poor weight shift senses that he is not stable and will often stop walking if there is a crowd around him or anyone who might inadvertently push into him. He has poor balance reactions and his trunk cannot lengthen and shorten as needed.

Learning good weight shift during stroke recovery is very important.

Does the trunk always move into elongation on the weight bearing side? No. Complex movements allow a person to vary how the trunk is bent or straightened, lengthened and shortened. A person can override the need to elongate on the weight bearing side if he uses more muscle strength or a varied body position to counterbalance his center of gravity moving beyond his base of support in that direction.

An example might be a man standing and reaching out four feet to the right side of his body with his right hand in order to grab an object at his knee level. In this case, the trunk will bend and not become longer on that side as the weight shifts.

Because he is bending over on the side he is shifting toward (his right), he may need to start lifting the left foot off the ground and out to the left to counterbalance the overextended movement to the right.

Not following Key #4 of elongation will require more effort to remain balanced. If he loses his balance to the right while doing this activity, he may even need to take a protective step with his left foot toward his right side.

Complex movements occur often such as in sports and on the job. They also occur even when we are cleaning the house or working outdoors in the yard. When a person has learned the normal weight shift pattern in Key #4, then these complex movements are much easier to coordinate.

Summary

In summary, these keys should help focus stroke recovery on relearning ways to move the body more normally.

Tapping into what the Hero has already spent a lifetime doing, should help to progress the level of function and safety during stroke recovery.

Chapter 5

"When It Comes to Learning Balance, How Low Can You Get?"

Balance begins on the floor where there is no fear of falling but ample opportunity to practice the right moves!

However, what happens on the floor does not stay on the floor! What is learned there will continue to be useful all the way up to standing and beyond!

When discussing normal movement patterns in this chapter we will eliminate any neurological or physical damage or problem in our study. We will look at how people move before a stroke.

Let's consider why the baby chose the movement that he did. Why did he keep using one way of moving and not continue the awkward movements? Furthermore, why have most humans around the world and throughout time decided as infants to use nearly the same ways to move?

These questions are important because the skills the brain learned in the School of Normal Movement as infant and small child were intact and making movement functional and fun. These skills served a stroke survivor well up until the time he had a stroke. Wouldn't it make sense to learn more about the way a person learned to move in the first place to help a stroke survivor recover some of those movement skills? The answer is simple. Yes.

The movements worked and they worked well. The brain is not silly!

The discovered movements were easy to perform, effective in reaching goals and efficient because they were less tiring than other ways that were tried! The skills were remembered by the brain and became automatic movements.

This is how we were made to move our body mass in the presence of gravity using muscles, bones and joints in order to stay balanced to the best of our ability!

A Study of Normal Movement

Let's start this study of normal movement!

Here we are on the floor! (*Photo A*)

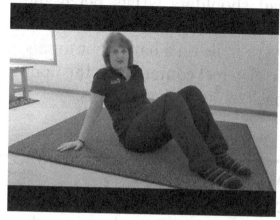

Photo A

Let's get lower! (*Photo B*)

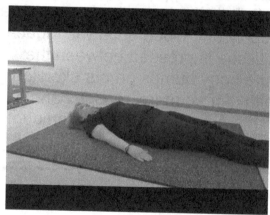

Photo B

This is the perfect position to get started with learning components of balance which will aid in performing normal movement.

If we lie on our back on the floor, we feel pressure at the back of the head, shoulders, wrists, pelvis and heels. These are the particular places we would feel discomfort if we were to lie on a hard floor for an extended time. We also feel contact with the floor along our spine, back of our legs and arms.

Side Note... but very important!

The pressure points are of particular interest for someone who cannot move themselves in bed because it is in these places the skin and what is under the skin will begin to breakdown. Sores can develop due to low blood supply in the compressed muscle and skin. Soft tissue in our bodies needs a constant blood supply and blood supply is reduced greatly when the tissue is pressed between the floor or bed and the bony bumps on our skeleton. Movement is healthy for so many reasons and reducing the risk of a pressure sore is paramount for good health!

To make rolling over easier, this person begins to lift her head and then look about halfway over to the side where she wants to roll. (*Photo C*)

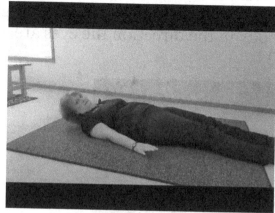

Photo C

This in turn will engage the far shoulder in the photo. She will then begin to lift that shoulder and the trunk on that side will begin to shorten as the shoulder and pelvis on that far side move toward each other. (*Photo D*)

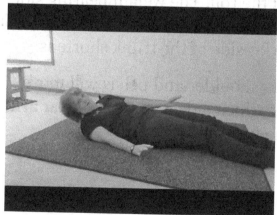

Photo D

She will lift the foot and not need to push herself off the floor with her far foot.

As the far arm lifts off the floor, the leg on the same side begins to lift, too. Both the arm and leg will begin to cross over the body in the direction the eyes are looking. (*Photo E*)

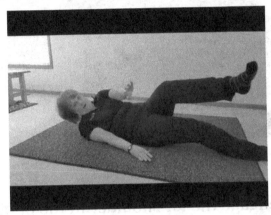

Photo E

This person's nearer arm remains flat on the floor. The body is shifting weight over to the nearer side which is in the direction of the roll. The weight bearing side (i.e. the nearer side), will elongate as it takes on more weight just as the far side of the trunk shortens.

Remember, the far shoulder and pelvis will move toward each other which aids in getting the far arm and leg up and the body turned.

This pattern continues until the body is halfway over to the tummy. The shoulder and pelvis on top are held closer to each other and that side of the trunk remains shortened to this point in the roll. (*Photo F*)

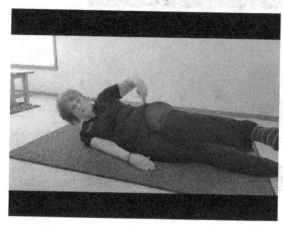

Photo F

Then things begin to change!

The changes that occur during the last part of the roll will be controlled, preventing a free fall over onto the tummy even though the body could easily flop over at this point.

The person's top leg is ready to start its descent to the floor and the arm will reach out and down until it touches the floor. (*Photo G*)

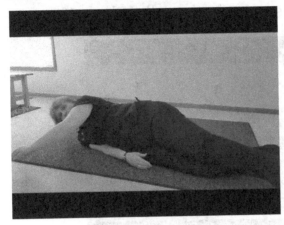

Photo G

What the shortened, upper side of the trunk does to accomplish this controlled descent to the tummy is to become slowly longer as the shoulder and pelvis begin to move away from each other on the way down to the floor.

That whole side of the body that had shortened now shifts back to the length it was before the roll. Observe the pelvis and shoulder on the shortened side spread out again to the distance they were before the roll. (*Photo H*)

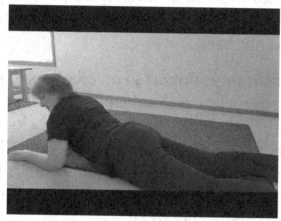

Photo H

The longer, lower side of the body which was carrying all the weight will also go back to its initial length at the end of the roll.

So once the body is over on the tummy, the trunk is again equal length on both sides.

Positioned on the tummy, this person is weight bearing on both elbows, the front of the pelvis, the knees and tops of the feet. She could be flat on the floor, too, but this example is a roll to resting on elbows which is a great position to do more functional activities involving the shoulders!

Bravo! The movement is complete!

Rolling from Tummy to Back

We aren't done with looking at this entire pattern yet because now we need to know what movements will get her back over onto her back.

From lying on her tummy supported on elbows she is in a good position to rock to one side and begin to unweight the nearer side in the photo. As she rocks to the far elbow on her right and she looks to her left. The side she looks toward is the side that initiates the roll. She will move the left side backward as she rolls over the right side of her body. (*Photo I*)

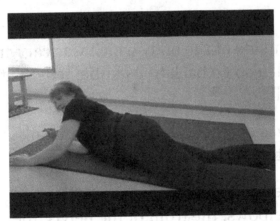

Photo I

The near side of her trunk begins to shorten as the far side lengthens and prepares for full weight bearing. Her head faces the shoulder that will again lift up against gravity only this time it lifts backward not forward as it did when she was on her back.

When she was rolling from her back to her tummy, she began turning her head toward what would become the longer or elongated weight bearing side. This time her head does not turn toward the side she will roll over, but rather toward the side she will lift.

Her head this time turns toward what will become the shorter side, the side that will be lifted up. Her head turns away from what will become the weight bearing side.

Simply put, when rolling she turns her head in the direction, she wants to either pull or push one shoulder up against gravity. Whichever side she lifts will become the shorter side of the trunk.

This is a key note because in therapy we do not want to be pushing or pulling on the shoulder to teach a person to roll. We need to find ways to encourage the brain to connect the head movement with the shoulder movement and then to the trunk movement. (*Photo J*)

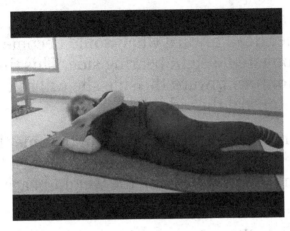

Photo J

The top side shortens as the lower side lengthens and takes on weight. The body rolls up onto its side.

Halfway over, both the upper and lower sides of the trunk reverse their movements of lengthening and shortening. (*Photo K*)

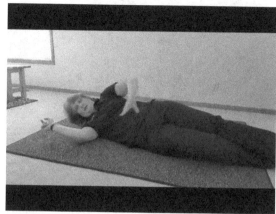

Photo K

The longer side shortens and the shorter side lengthens, both retuning to equal lengths by the time the body is weight bearing through both sides and she is again lying on her back. (*Photo L*)

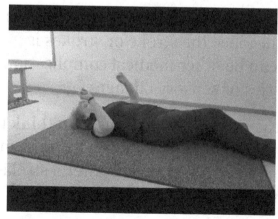

Photo L

We are back where we started! (*Photo M*)

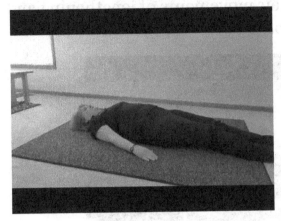

Photo M

Summary

We have gone back and looked at the kind of movement our brain was happy to do before a stroke. We have had a look at the Hero in our brain in action!

Who is your Hero?

Obviously, every stroke is different. The damage is different. The time since the stroke or strokes is different. There can be other medical complications, cognitive difficulties or sensory changes.

Strokes are not easy to understand, but I do think that there are those who perhaps without realizing it, may begin to think that the problems seen after a stroke begin in the arm or the leg instead of in the brain.

For them, the Hero seems to be in the poorly functioning limb and they can become upset with the arm or leg. They focus only on strengthening but it may not improve function.

I observe this at times when I see people participating in stroke recovery or exercises in the gym. Stroke survivors can become frustrated when trying to move with stiff arms and crazy legs. There are fingers that won't open, shoulders that won't lift, knees that won't bend and feet that twist.

The frustration is understandable. A stroke survivor is living with an arm or leg that just won't fully cooperate! These parts of the body seem to have a mind of their own!

What if they realized that their Hero is in their brain?

My desire as a physical therapist is to help clients reconnect their body with the Hero that is in their brain.

There are many questions.

Can your Hero help you no matter how much damage is caused by your stroke? Will the degree of damage influence the degree of recovery possible? How does anyone know how much recovery is left? Is there a ceiling to the degree of the recovery you can experience?

After years of treating stroke survivors, I can say that I do not know what can happen in any person's life, but I do know that the brain can continue to recover over time.

I look for signs of brain/body connection when I work with stroke survivors. These connections are easier to elicit in the early days and weeks after a stroke.

As time passes if the connections are not encouraged, the brain may begin to rely more and more on the side of the body that is not affected by stroke.

It can take more effort to force the brain to search for the muscles on the affected side and the stroke survivor has to be determined to try to move the affected side throughout the day when it is faster and easier to use the unaffected side.

For some there may be much more change possible. For others there may be less.

I would venture to say, though, that a stroke survivor would welcome any degree of further recovery that is possible. The time needed is anyone's guess.

A Word of Encouragement

We have taken a look back in this book at all of this nice, normal movement not with the intention of making you feel sad or discouraged. Regaining functional movement is not easy. It will take much concentration and determination along your journey!

Please remember that you are more than what you can do. Your personal value, who you are, is not based on your physical abilities.

There is a place for accepting what has happened and a place for working toward more recovery.

Every day is a day to be grateful for what we have and who we are. A grateful heart will put your heart at rest and ready to do what you can in that day regarding your stroke recovery.

As time continues after a stroke, progress can become slower. Some days it feels like maintaining range of motion and monitoring a good sitting position was all that was accomplished.

These two things in themselves are excellent ways to continue to leave the door open for more recovery.

Letting joints become stiff and never challenging poor attention to the stroke side of the body can lead to more limitations.

Be the person on the inside you want to be today. Add gratitude to your list of things to do! And enjoy your exercises as well as the people in your life!

If you would like further study of normal movement patterns used by your Hero for rolling, sitting up on the floor, getting up to hands and knees, shifting into kneeling and eventually standing up, then check out this online course! It is a wonderful supplement to this book!

Stroke Recovery Video Course:

Your Hero is in Your Brain

Link: strokewellness.com/herobrain

Chapter 6

"How Normal is Normal?"

Can a person's body move somewhat differently than we have described and still successfully roll from back to tummy? Of course.

There are slight variations between people. A person when rolling may lead more strongly with a shoulder or leg and less with her head, but all the movements will need to be present or the total movement will appear abnormal.

The question for us to consider is how the body moves after a stroke compared to how it moved before.

After a stroke can the head and shoulders and legs move like we have described in the previous chapter? Can the trunk sides shorten and lengthen to aid in maneuvers such as rolling or sitting up from the bed?

Let us experiment to see for ourselves if movement is easier when the body moves with these "normal movement patterns."

Suggestions for the Caregiver

Suggestion A

Here is an exercise. If you are not the stroke survivor, try the techniques pictured in the previous chapter. Then try variations such as rolling to your back by first picking up your leg without picking up your head, or roll back to your back by first trying to lift one side of your pelvis before you weight shift.

See for yourself if there are some ways that require less effort and others that require more.

Suggestion B

Now pretend you, as the caregiver, are a stroke survivor and try a few different ways to roll. Remember, in this exercise that only one side of your body moves on its own!

1. Only move your 'good' side and try to roll to either side.

2. Help your 'stroke' side with your 'good' side by grabbing the 'stroke' wrist or putting your 'good' foot under the 'stroke' foot before rolling.

3. Roll with your knees already bent and grab the 'stroke' wrist. Raise your arms up to the ceiling, turn your head toward your 'good' side and roll. Then do the same rolling toward your 'stroke' side.

4. Imagine learning how to raise your head and then your 'stroke' arm and leg like we talked about in the last chapter. How would it feel if the 'stroke' side of your trunk actually started to shorten as you rolled toward your 'good' side? You might need help for guidance initially but if you learned this, if your Hero could help you, how would that feel? Would it make this functional activity more fun?

Normal Movement - Is It Obvious?

The components of normal movement are obvious. How do I know this? You need no educational degree or special training to recognize normal movement. How do I know that?

Have you ever been sitting in a restaurant and watched people come in and take a seat? What caught your eye? Did you immediately notice if someone's movements were not 'normal'? How did you know these movements were not normal? (I ask these questions not to cause embarrassment to anyone who has a movement challenge, but only in discussing the existence of normal movement patterns.)

May I suggest that you were able to recognize the overall way the person moved and it looked more difficult, off center and less balanced or controlled?

Aha!

You may not be able to describe all the components necessary to create movement that looks normal to you, but you sure know when it isn't normal!

Side Note!

There is nothing "wrong" with the movements people use after a stroke or brain injury. Just getting up and moving and getting out again in public is fantastic!

Getting out can also have such a positive impact mentally because seeing new sights and socializing is refreshing! The purpose of this chapter is to encourage improved movement for the sake of enjoying easier movement and not meant in any way to make anyone feel self-conscious after a stroke.

In my professional opinion, stroke rehabilitation and recovery should be focused on releasing the Hero that is in your brain. That Hero made life so much easier for you before the stroke.

When the Hero in your brain is not reconnected well to your stroke side, orchestrating more fluid normal movement patterns is tough to do. What we end up noticing instead of fluid movements are movement struggles related to movement components that are missing.

Why Maintaining Joint Movement is Important

If muscles and joints do not move well for an extended time, but are fixed in place by tightness or dangle loosely with too much laxity, then changes can occur in muscles and joints that become structural and more permanent.

This means that even if the Hero gets better able to start controlling a joint, the actual structures of that joint may have become contracted or immovable. To prevent this, doing daily range of motion exercises and monitoring body position at rest are very important.

All types of movement may be necessary to maintain range of motion in the joints. This includes active movement, assisted movement and passive movement.

Setting Your Hero Up for Success

Best case scenario for stroke recovery... find, redevelop, reconnect and utilize the Hero that is in your brain as soon as possible.

A neuro physical or occupational therapist should be able to help guide you!

Your Hero is more than sheer balance and more than sheer strength. It is the entire movement process.

Your Hero calls to you from the past! Somewhere inside your brain is the memory of normal movement pattern components. The parts of the brain that make up your Hero can weave together all those lessons learned in infancy and those movements that you have enjoyed all your life.

Summary

I like to consider your Hero as a kind of movement memory in your brain but it takes focus, determination and time to find the pathways that lead from the Hero in your brain to your body.

Believe in your Hero and exercise into those movements that may be most difficult today.

Remember good movement can be fun and can give you so much joy!

Chapter 7

"Play it Again, Sam!"

There is something very interesting about play. Ready for it? It is FUN! That is the number one reason why anyone plays! Kids play games they think are fun. Adults play games that they think are fun!

When it comes to moving, the best way to get the best movement back is finding something that is fun and also has been experienced in the past! The brain opens up to exploring new pathways during play. The focus becomes the activity or game, not the specific movement. The brain looks around within itself to figure out how to weave together the combination of movements needed to do the game.

During play, the brain waits and longs to feel good. Play makes us feel happy.

When I am working with someone who has had a stroke, I use techniques to help normalize muscle tone or tenseness. I help prepare the limb or body to move.

I also begin to think about what kind of activity will encourage the components of movement I want to see the person using.

The hardest thing might be determining the kind of activity a particular person would like to do.

Balloons and Balls

I find that a balloon brings a smile to just about anyone's face. Once I get a balloon blown up and the person is in a safe position to begin to participate, I can soon use the placement of the balloon to encourage so many desirable arm and leg movements.

A great feature to balloon play is that balloons move slowly. They come in slowly toward someone giving that person time to plan (motor plan) how they will catch it or hit it. It floats.

The slow descent of a balloon means that the person has to hold a position and wait for the balloon to get there. That creates stability before mobility. Since holding shoulder positions is not always easy after a stroke, this gives the person a great opportunity to work on it.

Balloons are light. With a gentle push or tap a balloon will respond quickly and can travel far. Impacting something in the surrounding environment brings a sense of having some control. After months of being dependent and having limited impact on things, balloon play can create a brand new experience!

Note of caution: Be sure that those using balloons in therapy, the stroke survivor and anyone in the room, are not allergic to latex if the balloon is not latex free. Also do not leave balloons where unattended small children or toddlers or anyone with compromised cognitive ability could play with the balloon due to swallowing risks.

From balloons we can then graduate to a light bouncing ball. This kind of ball may require a quicker response, two handed maneuvering, the opening of fingers and hands as well as eye/hand control. A ball often helps to encourage rhythmic, anticipated movement so that the brain must work within a set timeframe.

There are endless ways to play with a balloon, inflatable beachball or ball. I have used bats, rackets, sticks and just the person's hands to bat at balloons or balls. I have used cups and upside down cones to catch a tossed ball.

By using an object in the hand, several goals can be reached. Hand grasp, arm swing, elbow extension, balance reactions and trunk movements can all be encouraged. How I use each thing in a session will depend on where I see the need for improving a specific normal movement pattern. I don't use play for random movements during a therapy session.

Play creates joy and helps someone feel better about himself and his circumstances. Depression often occurs with strokes. Play brings an added benefit of social interaction which can address some levels of depression.

Play in Therapy is Goal-Focused

I start out each therapy session with the goal in mind that I want to see some kind of new active movement that is controlled and meaningful. I encourage any kind of movement, but purposeful movement will make the greatest difference in recovery.

I have seen patients during even one session progress from needing total or maximum assistance in order to move a part of their body to being able to move a whole limb independently.

Therapy should always be goal-oriented! It takes much concentration and guidance, but when the connection to the body is made, the brain begins to do things it wasn't doing before. Goal-focused therapy is very satisfying.

Play can start out as a totally guided movement and can happen even if the activity must be done with the person lying on his side on a mat table. Perhaps someone has no sitting balance or it takes too much effort to maintain a sitting position. I may place a ball or balloon on the mat and give the person a goal as to where to push it or I may ask him to pick it up and specifically place it somewhere.

Slowly as I sense with my hands that the right muscles are engaging, I will lessen the help I am giving and allow the person to perform more and more of the activity on his own.

This activity may progress to doing the same things with the ball on an incline which means more force is needed to get the ball to roll up hill. It may progress from batting a balloon back and forth in side lying to doing it in sitting.

As the therapist, I am constantly thinking of the right kind of challenge and determining when to introduce a new movement or change the body position.

Summary

Some therapy techniques can feel like play. Play looks different at different stages of recovery. The good thing about this kind of therapy is that it is all done with a purpose in mind.

That purpose is getting back another component of normal movement that will enable the person to improve in other areas of life when, for instance, good shoulder, trunk or hip skill is required.

I love stroke rehab because it allows me to be creative and to engage the person in finding the Hero within! And besides that, play just makes everyone feel and move better!

Chapter 8

"Neuro Therapy"

In this book we have looked at ways a stroke survivor moved before a stroke. These same normal movements should continue to be the focus for stroke recovery even years after the stroke.

The kind of movements that are most functional are movements that align with normal movement patterns and once mastered will definitely be easier to do!

Not attaining full recovery of an arm or leg can be disappointing or frustrating for some and this book is not intended to highlight your limitations or struggles, but to encourage the best functional movement you are able to create.

The effects of a stroke are life changing for most people. Stroke recovery is not at all easy and we never know what will be the fullest degree of recovery possible.

As stated in the beginning of this book, learning about the Hero in your brain is meant to be an eye opener to help you choose the kind of therapy that will be most beneficial.

The overall emphasis of this book is to remind you that the stroke started in your brain and improving the brain's abilities to communicate with your body should be the target of a good stroke recovery program.

Muscles and joints are affected by a stroke, but to think that all one has to do is strengthen muscles will leave many people wondering why they lack the functional abilities for which they long.

One may wonder why the shoulder bunches up every time that arm is lifted or why the hand closes tightly when trying to put on a shirt. One may wonder why only focusing on dragging a foot forward in standing is not increasing safe, independent gait. There is a much bigger picture to consider.

Optimizing the outcome of rehab is important. Many stroke survivors work very hard to regain mobility and the use of an arm or hand.

Learning to move the body using more normal movement patterns which include proper weight shift as well as stability and mobility will help improve the quality of an activity. A better physical performance is the goal and it brings greater satisfaction.

Find the help you need. Recovery is a journey and often for a better outcome the help of a therapist who is skilled in neuro therapy can be the ticket to reaching your goals.

The Neuro Difference

Let's look at an example of orthopedic rehabilitation and neuro rehabilitation. Both are valuable!

If someone has had a total knee replacement, then therapy should focus on regaining all the available knee range that the surgery can offer. This will most likely include getting full extension of the knee and at least 110 degrees of knee bend, more is even better!

If these degrees of motion are reached and strength is recovered then the person should be able to walk and return to enjoyable activities and work.

The rate of recovery will differ because everyone's body tissues heal somewhat differently. Some people have more swelling and some people have more pain which may affect the rate of recovery. In the end, the hope is to gain good range of motion, good strength and a good walking pattern. These improvements of the injured site will be very visible!

In order to get a knee back to full range the therapist may use different techniques to influence the muscles, tendons and ligaments around the joint.

This may include instruction on using cold packs to help reduce swelling or putting the foot up on a chair or footstool to stretch the back of the knee. It may involve using a stationary bike to stretch the knee into more degrees of bend.

Throughout recovery the therapist will be giving the person exercises and instruction that will promote healing at the knee. It was the actual knee joint that was injured and replaced so this is where therapy is focused.

Now let's consider a stroke. The injury did not occur in the shoulder, hand or the knee. It occurred in the brain. The blockage or the bleed was medically treated and there was injury to the brain tissue.

The brain controls body movements and the ability to function in daily life. The effects of stroke are visible when we notice changes such as poor limb control, memory problems or speech difficulties. We don't see the actual damaged area in the brain unless we have medical imaging.

There is swelling in the brain, too, just as there would be swelling around an injured knee. However, in the case of stroke no one is really complaining that their brain looks different on one side or lacks 'range of movement'. Also, the body tissue around a knee is not like this type of injury. This is neural tissue made up of nerve cells in the brain and is nothing like the cells that make up tendon, bone and ligaments. It is a complex injury that directly affects multiple parts of the body because it is a neurological injury. Brain tissue is very specialized.

The brain is a control center. Because of that, areas of the brain that are affected by lack of oxygen (cell death) caused by the stroke will diminish the control of different areas of the body. If the damage is on the left side of the brain, diminished control is seen on the right side of the body.

Remember, the arm and leg did not lose control of themselves. Nothing in the arm or leg changed. The brain changed and lost the ability to control the arm or leg. Understanding this will help you in choosing the right kind of therapy!

The underlying feeling of someone who has had a stroke is loss of control because the control center has been injured.

Considerations for Good Stroke Recovery

Simply put, therapy should focus on loss of control from the brain down. It should be about learning to influence arm or leg movements by regaining the brain to body communication skills needed for muscle control. Control starts in the brain and goes to the muscles.

A spaceship can be very removed from the command center on earth, but the commands that are needed from the command center are vital for accomplishing the mission.

Cut or garble the communication and things go awry. The solution lies in improving the communication problem not fixing the spaceship which is not broken.

Restore useful communication and things are back on track. The spaceship did not break. t lost direction due to lack of control.

As time passes there can be secondary problems in the limb due to being poorly controlled by the brain. Muscles and tendons can become very stiff and joints that are not stretched can change.

Braces may be necessary to maintain good joint positions.

The appropriateness and fit of each brace should be reevaluated often by the therapist. The goal of therapy is to reduce the need of bracing or to lighten the control of the brace as the joint or body area control improves. Examples of when braces are used:

- Maintaining the correct bend in the ankle so that a person can weight bear on that foot and practice hip and knee control.

- Maintain an open hand so that the palm can be washed to prevent infection and also so the hand can have the opportunity to regain the ability to grasp a cup.

Joint changes after a stroke are secondary problems due to the loss of the brain's control. These problems are not the primary problem which happened at the injured site.

These changes, though, can further complicate recovery because even if the brain over time starts sending the right message to that area of the body, the structural changes of the joint may not allow the muscles to move the joint normally.

This is why it is important to keep tight joints stretched and vulnerable, lax joints protected from injury.

Also, over time, if abnormal movement patterns are not changed and are practiced over and over again by the brain then these less functional patterns become very strong pathways of communication between the brain and body.

This emphasizes the importance of gaining good shoulder and hip control early in the rehab process because good use of these particular joints will affect the use of the hand and the quality of walking.

Abnormal movement patterns that go unchanged limit how functional an arm or leg can be. The synergistic pattern becomes engrained making it hard to convince your brain to look for a better pathway.

An example of this is when the shoulder is continuously lifted up toward the ear when the person raises his arm and years later this same pattern keeps him from being able to get his hand above his head.

Making changes to these abnormal or compensatory pathways becomes more difficult over time than it would have been if they were addressed closer to the time of the stroke. Early intervention is always best.

Habits are always hard to change but not impossible to change! As time passes, progress can still be made though it may certainly become slower and will take a lot of determination.

When a person is able to change the functional use and control of their hand, he needs to consciously continue to use this new skill all the time throughout his day, not just when he is practicing an exercise.

The goal is to begin to see the hand used more automatically and naturally during normal tasks.

I sometimes see a patient working very hard during the therapy session to master a great, new movement, but when the session ends that person goes right back to favoring the use of the good side!

It is far better to incorporate using the stroke side throughout the day whenever you can so that it becomes more automatic for the brain to choose to use it.

One type of therapy is to restrict the use of the unaffected arm for 30 minutes by wrapping it against the trunk with a bedsheet. The person will not be able to use the unaffected arm at all. The affected arm is placed on a table and a simple activity is set up such as reaching for an object. The brain is forced during this time to only think about the affected side as it contemplates doing the activity.

This activity can help open up new brain pathways to the affected side.

The Neuro Approach - Billions of Cells are Able to Make New Pathways

Let's consider these sensory questions:

- How can sensory motor input at the shoulder during therapy help the brain start communicating with the shoulder like it did before the stroke?

- How does the brain use those sensations to promote the kind of active movement it had before the stroke?

- How can improving the position of the shoulder result in changed muscle tone so that the tone becomes more like it was before the stroke?

- How can the feel of the shoulder and arm being moved through a normal movement pattern affect the brain's ability to 'find' the shoulder, use or move it for a familiar task and possibly even remember that movement the next day?

In short, how can the brain recognize and reproduce the normal movement patterns it had before the stroke?

If you go back and visit a place from your childhood, perhaps your old elementary school or neighborhood, and there is still someone there who recognizes you who knew you well then, communication is soon very easy!

Sensory and motor input to the brain triggers the movement memory. Add active movement after passive sensory input for that movement and the brain finds ways to connect sensory to motor. It is called sensory motor movement and that is how everyone moves.

Knock out sensation in a limb and the brain often cannot learn to move that limb again. Movement and the sensation of that movement are tied closely together.

Summary

After a stroke, your Hero remembers how you previously moved your body. The brain can remember successful movement patterns it used before the stroke.

The parts of the brain that were involved in laying down a foundation of effective, efficient and easy movement patterns so many years ago still have connections in your brain. Those connections may be weak but they are still there.

Maximize these connections and build new pathways! Does this mean anyone and everyone can fully recovery after a stroke? No.

Your brain is injured and you may not be able to get back your movement fully (though some do very well in rehabilitation).

Do we know when someone has reached their fullest recovery? No.

For this reason, I advise you to consider working with a neuro therapist for as long as you can. Even to be reevaluated once or twice a year for further recommendations can be very helpful in gaining optimal recovery.

Chapter 9

"Where Do I Go from Here?"

What Can You Do to Encourage Continued Recovery after a Stroke and What are Your Rehab Options?

There are ways to continue to optimize recovery and function. It starts with maintaining good range of motion and decreasing the risk of any injury to the body. It continues with making sure you are moving both sides of your body every day.

Try to find ways to communicate with your Hero. Exercise in the best way possible through brain-focused neuro therapy.

This book offers some suggestions for better movement patterns to include in your therapy and was written in order to help open your eyes to the kind of stroke rehabilitation that will aid you in your journey!

Seek out the kind of therapy that speaks to your Hero and discover brain-focused, targeted exercises to relearn joyful, everyday movement!

Physical Therapists are educated in the science of movement and neuromuscular reeducation. They are movement specialists and are clinically trained to medically monitor stroke survivors through extensive exercise programs.

Physical Therapists and Occupational Therapists can offer recommendations for assistive devices, bracing and home modifications.

Stroke survivors should be assisted to transition from the hospital to the rehabilitation center and then from home life to community level activities.

After returning home, the therapist can help the stroke survivor determine realistic and specific goals for returning to their family life, community life, leisure activities and sometimes even back to work.

Can I Keep Working with a Physical Therapist for Wellness Exercise after Insurance Ends?

Many physical therapists are now offering private pay sessions for ongoing exercise and movement recovery for stroke survivors after insurance stops paying. In some cases, telehealth visits on the computer can be very helpful in maintaining a good exercise program!

Some therapists have clinics and some offer convenient in- home personal wellness sessions even when someone is no longer homebound. Private pay therapists are not restricted by insurance guidelines that require discharging before personal goals are met, nor do these therapists need to diminish the frequency of service due to slower progress.

The stroke survivor sets the goals they want to achieve and the therapist works with him toward reaching these goals.

Many people across the USA appreciate the primary care of physical therapists without the need for a physician's referral. Physical therapists can now be directly accessed in most states for the evaluation of neuromuscular and musculoskeletal disorders.

Direct access reduces cost and reduces the wait time for getting started with the appropriate therapist.

Depending on the state, private pay therapy may not need a physician's referral for several weeks to a few months after the evaluation.

Your therapist can work closely with your physician to make sure any medical concerns are promptly addressed. Physicians are delighted that their patients can receive on-going, effective, medically-based rehabilitation.

Telehealth PT

A new area of stroke care is telehealth physical therapy. The therapist meets the client in online video consultations to evaluate and treat musculoskeletal injury, set up and maintain wellness programs and offer valuable education about the client's situation. Caregivers for neurologically impaired loved ones can gain valuable professional support.

The telehealth platform selected should be on a secure site. Ask your therapist what platform they are using to be sure the video call is secure and your privacy is protected.

Online sessions are definitely time efficient and convenient. Imagine no travel time to and from the clinic. It eliminates the wait time in the waiting room. Appointments can also be made early in the day and later into the evening which is helpful for busy people. Clients can also avoid the walk into the clinic from the parking lot in adverse weather or when walking is challenging.

Understand the Qualifications of Your Rehabilitation Professional

Physical therapists earn university or college degrees and pass a national board exam to qualify for a license to practice. Each state issues their own physical therapy license and has their own practice act that the therapist must follow.

Physical Therapists study advanced rehabilitative medical education combining in-depth study of anatomy, physiology, pathology, pharmacology, neurology, diagnostic imaging, prosthetics, statistics, medical equipment, wound care, massage and myofascial release, manual therapy, gait analysis, kinesiology, therapeutic exercise and more.

Before graduating, they must practice under clinical supervision in various health care settings for months and demonstrate competent skills. (Settings include nearly all hospital departments, home health, outpatient, schools, skilled nursing facilities, and rehab centers.)

It is mandatory to maintain set levels of continuing education throughout their career in order to remain licensed.

Personal trainers, massage therapists and other exercise specialists can also assist after a stroke and can inform you about their level of training, expertise and accountability.

Feel free to ask to see your provider's license, certificates and credentials for the work or service you receive.

In summary, direct access to physical therapy is available in most states this means you do not need to get a physician's referral before calling to make an appointment to see a physical therapist. However, each state is governed by its own physical therapy practice act so ask the therapist what they need from you before you go to your appointment.

As you choose your stroke recovery partner(s) (therapists, coaches, personal trainers...) *ask and understand how each one is trained to help you!*

Conclusion

I have written about the Hero that is in your brain because I want you to better understand that a stroke is a brain injury and that is where therapy needs to begin.

I want you to become your own best advocate during your journey of recovery. I want you to recognize good neuro therapy and to realize that recovery does not necessarily have to end when insurance ends.

No one else wants your freedom of movement, independence and functional use of your body, more than you do! Find others who will support you in this and help you reach your goals. *Those goals are uniquely yours!*

I trust that you are beginning to understand how best to approach your recovery from the brain down. You will be much more satisfied with the quality of your movement if you do!

You will experience safer mobility when your body begins to function more like it did before your stroke because the brain has gained better control.

Remember, this book is not an exercise book but it should lead you to a greater understanding of the kind of exercises that will be most helpful and will help to release the Hero that is your brain!

I encourage you to find help from professionals who understand the medical effects of stroke as well as ways to safely promote your personal goals, optimize outcome, improve your function and address your mobility needs so you can be doing things you love to do.

Never lose sight of your goals and remember to be grateful each and every day!

Wishing you a lifetime of new discoveries!